ABS!

50 of the best core exercises to strengthen, tone, and flatten your belly

Ideal for all levels of fitness.

Howard Allan VanEs, M.A.

D0814415

Letsdoyoga.com Wellnes ~~Series~~

Published by

letsdoyoga.com

Howard VanEs, Publisher
4651 Antelope Way
Antioch, CA 94531
415-309-1290
www.letsdoyoga.com
info@letsdoyoga.com

Disclaimer

The information and exercises in this booklet are not intended to diagnose or treat any health condition. If you are not currently exercising it is advisable to seek to seek the advice of a physician before embarking on any program of physical exercise.

If you have an ulcer or any other serious stomach problem DO NOT perform any of these exercises. If any exercise produces pain, immediately STOP and skip that exercise.

Free Wellness Newsletter

As a service to our readers Letsdoyoga.com publishes a wellness newsletter. This monthly newsletter features articles and ideas to help you live a happier and healthier life as well as insights, tips and ideas to deepen the practice of yoga. If you would like to receive a copy of Yoga Health and Wellness Newsletter visit **www.letsdoyoga.com** and enter your email address.

Acknowledgements

Letsdoyoga.com would like to acknowledge and thank the following people whose contribution was integral to the production of this book:

Designer: Howard Petlack, hpetlack@agoodthingink.com

Photographer: Karen Margroff Dunn, KMDPortraits.com

Model: Lois Kaye Pope, contact her in care of info@letsdoyoga.com

Location: The Yoga and Movement Center, Walnut Creek, CA
Diane Valentine, Director www.yoga-movement.com

Letsdoyoga.com offers seminars and workshops on the following wellness related topics:

Stress management

Office ergonomics

Insomnia

Anxiety

Tight shoulders

Back care

Abdominal exercises

Meditation

Pranayama (yogic breathing)

Secrets of stretching

Various Yoga oriented workshops

If you are interested in having any of the above trainings presented to your organization please contact Howard VanEs at:

info@letsdoyoga.com or 415-309-1290.

Lack of activity destroys the good condition of every human being, while movement and methodical physical exercise save it and preserve it."

—Plato

Table of Contents

Foreward

Congratulations on purchasing this book for exercising your abdominal muscles. You have taken an important step in improving the quality of your health and lifestyle.

As you may already know there are tremendous benefits to exercise including the controlling and prevention of chronic conditions such as cholesterol, blood sugar, blood pressure and metabolic syndrome; the slowing or reversing of such common ailments like arthritis, low back pain and pre-menstrual syndrome, as well as helping to control emotional conditions like mild depression. And while it true that working your abdominals can help produce a trim, sexy mid-section what is also worthwhile realizing is that there are many other valuable benefits to having strong abdominals.

Strong abdominals help to minimize back pain, which is the number one reason for emergency room visits in the U.S. and tops the list for lost pay due to absenteeism. A well toned mid-section helps to improve posture while sitting and standing. For those individuals with desk jobs, this is critical to long-term comfort. Strong abdominal muscles also help to improve the athletic performance of sports enthusiasts at any level. And perhaps most importantly, strong abdominals increase one's overall quality of life. Think about it, everything from standing up, reaching, getting up and down off the floor or playing with the children become easier with strong abdominals. Finally, working your abs typically will result in a thinner, more toned body, which is good for one's self-esteem because you will feel more attractive.

Unfortunately, for many people a gap exists between wanting strong abdominals and attaining them simply because they don't know what exercises to do and how to do them. Long gone are the days of our elementary school sit-ups! In this book, yoga expert Howard VanEs will lead you through over 50 abdominal exercises that are categorized by easy, moderate, and challenging. You get great exercises for all four major groups of abdominal muscles. When you purchase this book, you can begin a routine that meets your fitness level while having many options to continuously challenge yourself, further increase your abdominal strength, and start enjoying the many benefits that come from having a well toned mid-section.

Once again, congratulations!

> *In good health,*
> Casey Conrad
> FOUNDER, THE TAKE IT OFF WEIGHT LOSS PROGRAM
> AUTHOR, WINNING THE STRUGGLE TO BE THIN

FREE bonus audio for readers of this book!

Go to www.abandstomachexercises.com/ free-audio-2 to get a "Yoga for Strong Core" workout audio.

About the Author

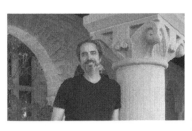 **Howard VanEs, M.A.** ERYT-500, has been committed to wellness and fitness for over 26 years. He has a deep passion for wellness, and a desire to help people learn about the many ways they can improve the quality of their health and lives through mind/body methods. His experience includes weight training, martial arts, yoga, stress management training, and work from his previous role as a psychotherapist. For over 20 years, Howard has been a dedicated practitioner of hatha yoga and has been teaching yoga for the last 16 years in the Bay Area of California.

Howard is the author of *Ageless Beauty & Timeless Strength* and is the primary author and editor of the Letsdoyoga.com wellness book series: *Beginning Yoga: A Practice Manual, Abs!, Tight Shoulder Relief* and co-author of *Office Ergonomics, Preventing Repetitive Motion Injuries and Carpal Tunnel Syndrome*. He is also the co-producer of the audio CD, *Shavasna/Deep Relaxation*, and creator of the *Yoga on Demand* audio program which features over 14 yoga audios. In addition to writing about and teaching yoga, Howard also leads yoga teacher trainings, wellness seminars and retreats worldwide.

His websites are:

www.letsdoyoga.com
www.exercisesforupperbody.com
www.agelessbeautybook.com
www.abandstomachexercises.com

Twitter: HowardVanEs@yogaman108
Email: info@letsdoyoga.com

FREE, bonus audio download!
Go to www.abandstomachexercises.com/ free-audio-2
to get a "Yoga for Strong Core" workout audio.

Major benefits of having toned abdominal muscles:

Improves digestion and elimination: The process of peristalsis (food moving through the digestive track) is greatly improved when you practice ab and stomach exercises. This is due to the actual movement of the exercise itself as well as improving the overall function of the organs and tissues associated with digestion. Elimination is also improved.

Reduces back pain/ protects the back: Weak abs put unnecessary strain on your lower back both in just holding your spine in a good stable posture as well as for everyday movements like bending over to pick something up getting in and out of a car. You need strength in your core to do this without hurting your back. Having strong abs also helps to reduce or eliminate lower back pain.

Improves athletic performance: Most movement begins with the core. Having toned abdominals helps your entire body function optimally. When you regularly practice ab and stomach exercises you will dramatically increase endurance and power through out your entire body. A strong core will also help protect you from injury during athletic activities.

Good posture: Strong abs help you keep good posture which means that your spine I more likely align properly. This improves the functioning and movement of your entire body as well as your nervous system.

Improves your breathing: The more toned your abs are the more they can assist in breathing. Try this little experiment. Sit upright in a chair and place your hands on your belly. Take a slow deep inhalation and then a long slow exhalation. Notice how your belly moves out on the inhalation and out on the exhalation. What makes these movement possible are your abs.

Helps maintain proper functioning of the stomach organs: When you exercise your abdominal area, the organs of this area get an internal massage. The organs are squeezed and soaked in fresh blood. In yoga this is referred to as a "tonifying" effect on the organs. Metabolic wastes are squeezed out and fresh blood with oxygen and nutrients are brought back into the organs.

Helps with pregnancy/child birth: Exercising before pregnancy as well as during pregnancy will make for easier child birth. It will also help your reduce stress, help keep you healthy and after you give birth, your body will return to its original form a lot quicker! Note: There are many stomach exercises that should be avoided or modified during pregnancy. Working with a knowledgeable fitness professional is highly recommended until you know which exercises to include and which to avoid.

Increases muscle mass: Challenging any muscle group with resistance exercises will build muscle. This is highly desirable not only for strength, but because the more muscle you have on your body the more calories you will burn, even at rest!

Enhances overall looks: Working your abs helps to flatten your belly and adds to a long lean look. If you watch your diet and add some exercise then you might just find your 6-pack too! By including ab and stomach exercises in your workout you probably burn more calories too. And when you look good and feel good, your self-confidence and self-esteem can soar!

Prevent hernias: Hernias are often caused by weak abdominal muscles. Simply put, strong abs will greatly decrease your chances of developing a hernia.

Less pressure on your joints: Having a strong core helps to stabilize your body. This keeps your body balanced and unwanted pressure off your joints, which can lead to injury and pain.

Improves your energy: According to some eastern practices the stomach is the seat of will power and making sure that this area is strong, flexible and healthy will allow energy to flow properly. Test this out for yourself. Do ten minutes of ab and stomach exercises and notice how your energy level improves!

About "six packs"

It is important to keep in mind that for most people exercise alone will not result in washboard abs. It is generally a combination of proper diet and exercise that produces a lean body and "six pack" abs. For your abdominals to show, a very low amount of body fat is needed. And there is a strong genetic component associated with this as well. So it may be extremely difficult for some people to have their abdominal muscles show. Not impossible, but quiet difficult. Keep in mind that only a very small (read tiny) percentage of the population has "wash board abs". Don't let this discourage you though from working your abs. As mentioned before there are tremendous benefits that come from working your abs. And if you exercise your abdominals properly, as part of an overall program of fitness and nutrition, then you will look great and feel good too. And who knows, you might just find your "six pack".

Abdominal Muscles

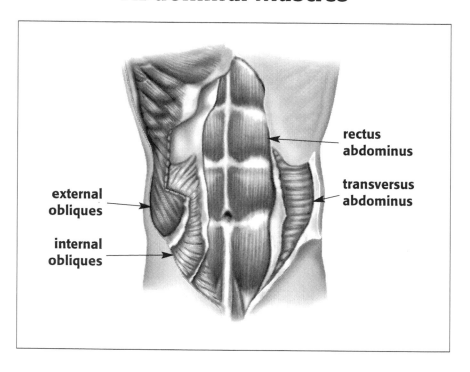

external
obliques

internal
obliques

rectus
abdominus

transversus
abdominus

Anatomy of abdominal muscles

"The primary functions of the abdominal muscles are to stabilize your body, keep the abdominal organs in place and to bear down in movements such as child birth, coughing, elimination, etc."

1. The outermost layer of the abdominal muscles is the rectus abdominis. When this muscle shows it is commonly referred to as a 6 pack. It runs from the pubic bone to the breast bone and middle ribs. The primary function of the rectus abdominis is flexion of the torso and also assists other muscles in compressing the abdomen.

2. The next layer of muscles are the internal and external obliques. These muscles run diagonally on the sides of the torso from the top of the hips to the middle ribs. Their primary function is twisting, side bending and rotation of the trunk. They also assist in flexion of the trunk.

3. The transversus abdominis is the deepest layer of abdominal muscle. This muscle goes around

the midsection - front to back with fibers run-
ning side to side. The lower portion attaches to
hip area (front and back) and the upper portion
attaches to the to the lower ribs. Contraction of
the transverse muscles pulls the belly in. These
muscles are more associated with autonomic
nervous system functions such as coughing,
bearing down, elimination and childbirth. An
easy way to connect with these muscles is to
place your hands on the sides of your of your
abdominal area and cough.

How to use this book

The abdominal exercises listed below are fall in into three levels of challenge: Easy, Moderate and Challenging. Each exercise is marked accordingly. If your mid-section hasn't had any exercise in a while then start with the exercises marked easy. Start with five to ten minutes three to four times a week. After a few weeks this will start to feel easy—at that point start adding a few moderate ones. If you have an exercise program of some sort then start with a few easy exercises to get warmed up and move to the moderate ones. Ten to twenty minutes three to five times a week would be good for you.

Once you have developed some ease with the moderate section start adding challenging exercises. And if you have a vigorous exercise program and are already doing some abdominal work start with a few of the easy exercises, a few moderate ones and then add the challenging ones. Twenty to thirty minutes three to five times a week will be ideal.

You'll find good variety of exercises for each level of challenge. Keep changing the ones you do — so your muscles are always being challenged and you don't get bored.

When your are finished exercising your abdominal muscles it is a good idea to stretch them out to rest. You will find a recommendation for this under the cool down section at the end of this book.

Increasing intensity

As you progress with your workouts you'll most likely want to make them more challenging. To increase intensity experiment with these ideas:

Repeat exercises

Shorten the rest period in between exercises

Add repetitions

Perform exercises in groups of 2-5 exercises-one right after another

Combine one or all of the ideas above!

"Remember, if something hurts don't do it!"

You see, you don't get old from age, you get old from inactivity, from not believing in something.

—Jack LaLanne

Standing fire wash
Level: easy

Stand with your legs a little wider than hip width apart and bend your knees. Place your hands on your thighs, with the baby-finger sides of your hands facing away from you. As you exhale completely, draw your belly button towards your spine. Holding your breath "out" pump your belly in and out up to 15 times. DO NOT let your self get out of breath and do not force yourself. In the beginning your may only be able to pump your belly 5 times. Work up to 2–3 rounds of 15 pulls over the course of a few weeks or months. This exercise is also good for improving your digestion.

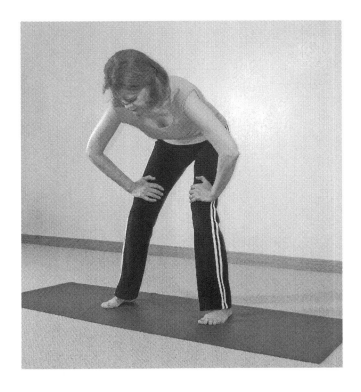

Woodchopper
Level: easy

Start by taking your feet 2 ½ to 3 feet apart. Interlace your fingers and take your hands up overhead. As you exhale bring your hands between your legs as if you were chopping wood. Now take your arms back up over head. Repeat 6 to 10 times. If you have any lower back issues be sure to bend you knees slightly. If for any 'reason this exercise hurts your back don't do it.

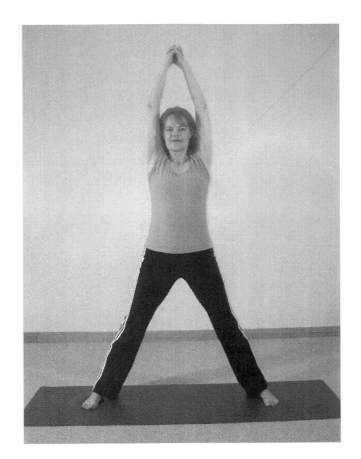

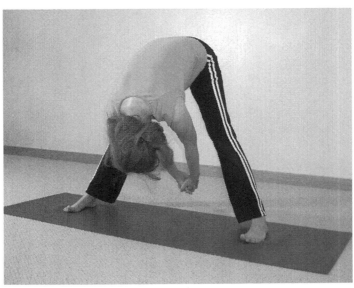

Woodchopper with one hand
Level: easy

This is just like the last version of Woodchopper except you only use one arm. For this version you will need a foam yoga block or a light book. Stand with you feet 2 1/2 to 3 feet apart. Holding the block or book in your right hand and take it up overhead. Keep your left arm and hand by your side. As you exhale take your right hand down between your legs. Now bring your right arm back up overhead. Repeat 3–5 times on the right and 3–5 times on the left.

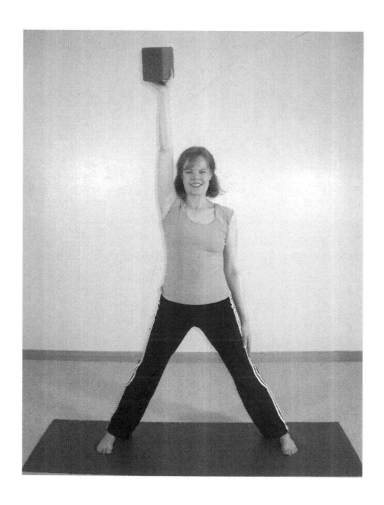

Standing bicycle
Level: easy

Begin by standing with your legs directly under your hips. Next interlace your fingers behind your head. As you exhale lift your left knee toward your stomach and bring your right elbow to the outside of your left knee. Release your left foot to the floor, lift your torso and your right elbow back up behind your head. Now do the other side bringing your right knee towards your stomach and your left elbow to the outside of your right knee. Go back to the right side and do 3–5 more rounds alternating sides as you perform the exercise.

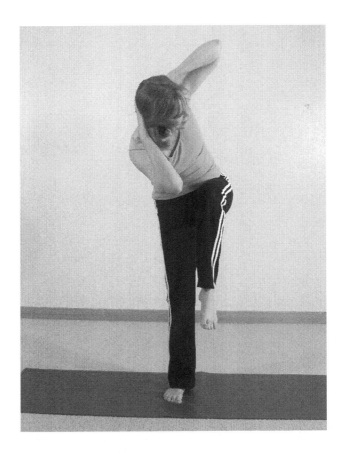

Get up, get down
Level: moderate

Begin by lying down on your back with your legs extended in front of you. Place a foam yoga block, book, or light dumbbell in your right hand and extend it straight up towards the ceiling. Keeping your right arm extended the whole time, bend your knees, place your feet on the floor and stand up in one smooth motion. Use your left hand to help you get up if need be. You should end standing on your feet with your right arm extended overhead. Now lay back down again onto the floor. Repeat 3–5 times and then do the other side. In addition to working the abs you'll also find this exercise to be very aerobic!

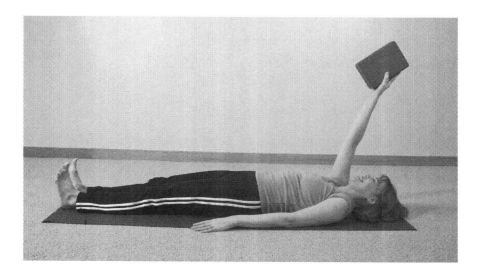

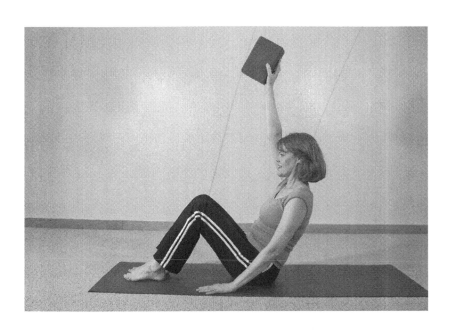

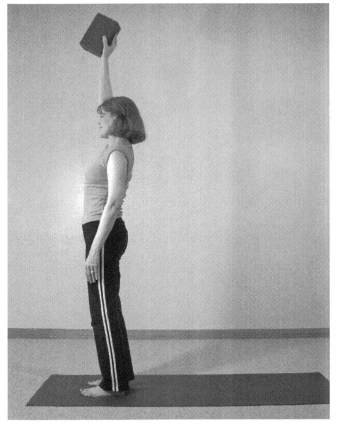

Seated row
Level: moderate

Start by sitting on the floor with both legs extended straight in front of you. Bring your arms to shoulder height, so that they are parallel to the floor and extend through your fingers.

Stretch into your heels and curl your torso back towards the floor a little. Keep reaching into your heels and your hands as you come up to an upright position, reaching towards your feet. Once again curl back towards the floor – this time going a little further and then come up as you just did. The further back you go, the more challenging the exercise. It is up to you. Do not go back any further than the lower tips of your shoulder blades, as it will be very difficult to get back up. Repeat the exercise 5–10 times.

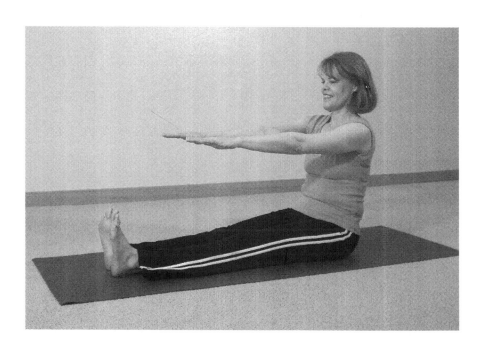

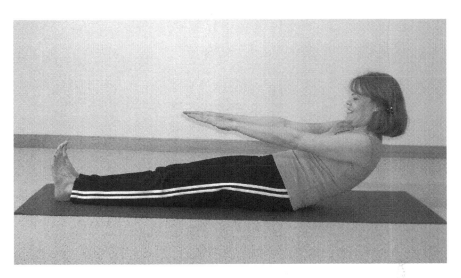

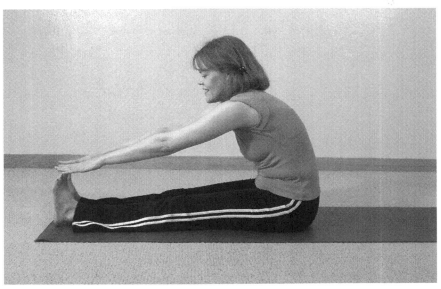

Easy Boat
Level: easy

Sit on floor with your knees bent and feet on the floor. Place your hands on the backs of your thighs and let your weight shift backwards slightly so that you are balancing just behind your sitz bones. Bring your shins parallel to the floor. Lift up through your spine. Hold for a slow count of 5 to 10.

Note: Your torso and legs should form a 45% angle.

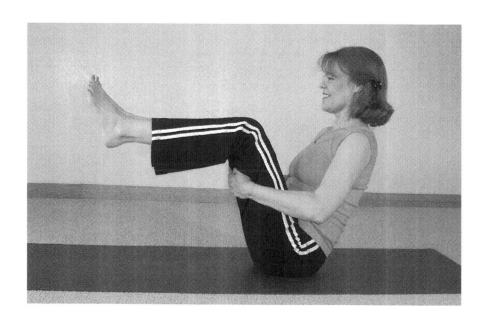

One Legged Boat
Level: easy

Sit on floor with your knees bent and feet on the floor.
Place your hands on the backs of your thighs and let
your weight shift backwards slightly so that you are
balancing just behind your sitz bones. Keeping your left
foot on the ground extend your right leg straight. Press
though your right foot and lift up through your spine.
Extend your arms so they are parallel to the floor. Hold
for a count of 5 and repeat with the left leg.

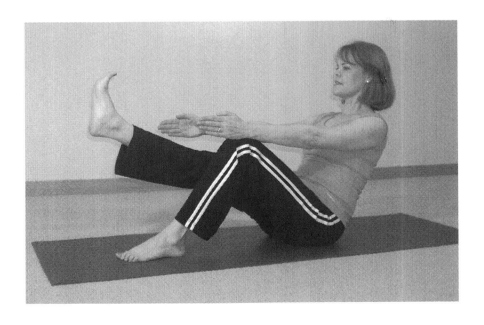

Boat
Level: moderate

Begin by sitting on floor with your knees bent and feet
on the floor. Place your hands on the back of your thighs
and let your weight shift backwards slightly so that you
are balancing just behind your sitz bones. Bring your
shins parallel to the floor. Extend your arms so they are
parallel to the floor. Your torso and legs should form a
45% angle approximately. Now extend both legs and
press through your feet and lift up through your spine.
You want your toes to be a little higher than your eyes.
Hold for a slow count of 5–10.

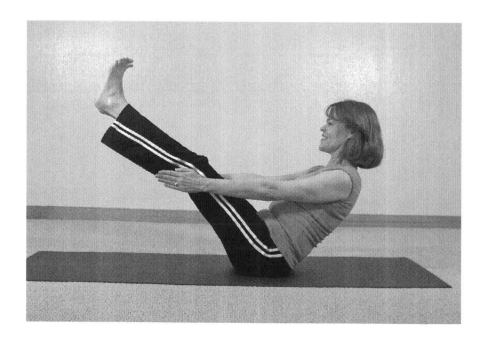

Boat with alternating knee to chest
Level: moderate

Begin by sitting on floor with your knees bent and feet on the floor. Place your hands on the back of your thighs and let your weight shift backwards slightly so that you are balancing just behind your sitz bones. Bring your shins parallel to the floor. Extend your arms straight so they are parallel to the ground. Lift up through your spine. Extend both legs and press through your feet and lift your torso up. Your torso and legs should form a 45% angle. Now, keeping your right leg extended, bring your left knee in towards your chest. Pause for a second and then extend your left leg as your bring your right knee in towards your chest. Repeat this cycle several times, making it as smooth as possible.

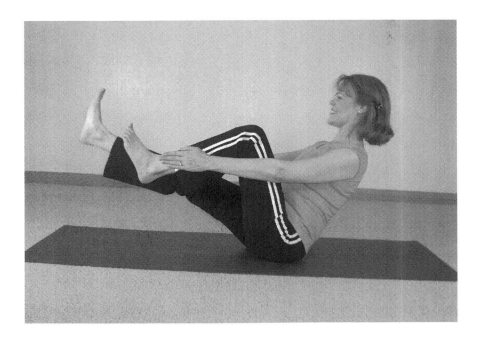

Challenging Boat
Level: challenging

Begin by sitting on floor with your knees bent and feet on the floor. Place your hands on your thighs and let your weight shift backwards slightly so that you are balancing just behind your sitz bones. Bring your shins parallel to the floor. Extend your arms straight so they are parallel to the ground. Lift up through your spine.

Now, interlace your fingers behind your head with your elbows out to the sides. Release your torso and legs towards the floor so that your feet are approximately 8–10" from the ground and your feet are just a little higher than your head. Hold for a count of 5–10. Carefully release to the floor on an exhale.

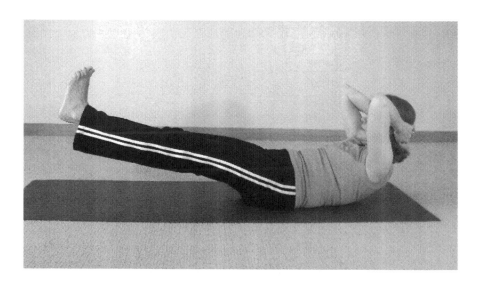

Leg spread
Level: moderate

Begin by sitting on the floor with your knees bent to the sides and the soles of your feet facing each other. Wrap your index fingers and middle finger around the inside of your big toes. (Alternately you can hold your ankles which will be very helpful if you have tight hamstrings).

Now, holding your big toes or ankles rock back just behind your sitz bones to balance. Lift your shins parallel to the floor while continuing to hold your toes or ankles. Start to spread and straighten your legs. Lift up through your torso and press into your feet. Hold for a slow count of 5–10 and release your hands and then feet to the floor.

Note: Be careful of what is behind you in case you fall backwards. Be sure to practice this exercise away from a wall.

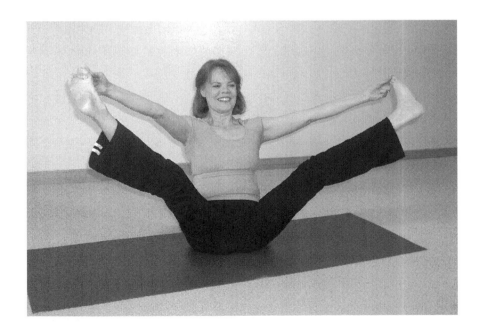

Follow the leader
Level: moderate

Begin by lying on your back with your knees bent and feet on the floor. Place your hands on your thighs. As you exhale press your belly button towards your spine, lift your torso and bring your chin towards your chest. Now take your right arm up over head behind you and at the same time bring your right knee into your chest. Imagine that a string was attached between your right knee and hand. Release your arm forward towards your knee and place your right foot back on the ground, letting your right hand rest on your thigh. Then do the left side —going back and forth from side to side. Focus on making the movement smooth. Repeat the entire cycle several times.

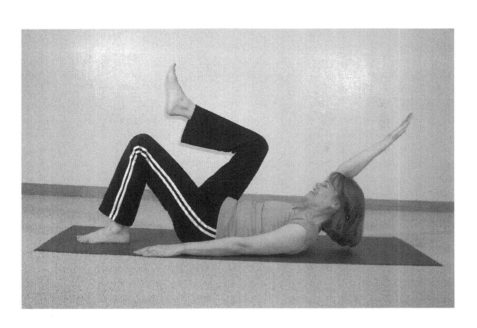

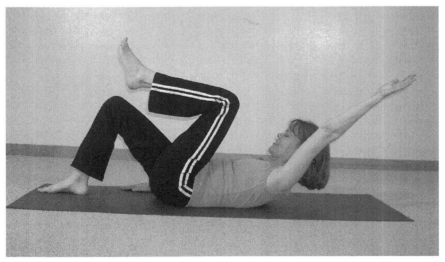

Leg circles
Level: easy

Begin by lying on your back. Bring your knees into your chest and extend your legs towards the ceiling. Separate your legs approximately 12" apart. Begin to make small circles with each leg moving independently (that is to say that your legs move out to the sides, away from head, together and then back towards head.) Repeat three times. Take your legs a little wider which will make your circles larger. Repeat three times again. Now make your circles even wider. Repeat three times. Now reverse direction of your circles and make them a little smaller. Repeat three times and make your circles even smaller. Repeat three times and then rest.

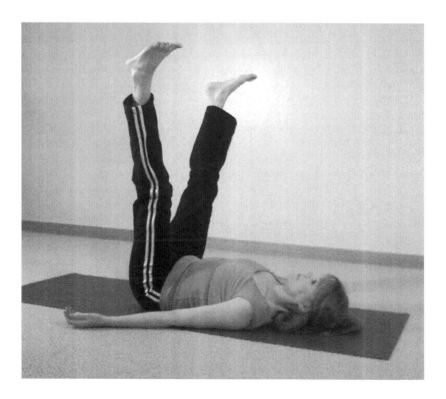

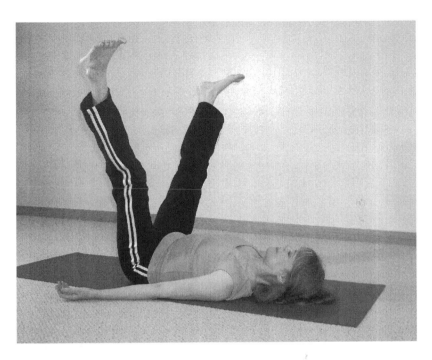

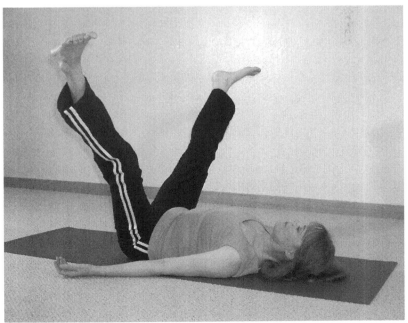

Reverse crunch
Level: moderate

Begin by lying on your back. Bring your knees into your chest and extend your legs up towards the ceiling. Extend your arms along side of your torso so that your hands are along side of your hips, palms down on the floor. As your inhale, press your hands into the floor and lift your hips—curling your tailbone upwards. As you exhale and lift your head and chest, and press your belly button towards your spine. Hold for 3–5 seconds and release. Repeat 3–5 times.

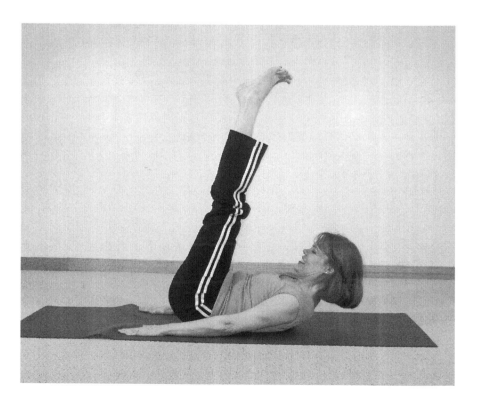

Reverse crunch - arms extended
Level: challenging

Begin by lying on your back. Bring your knees into your chest and extend your legs up towards the ceiling. Extend your arms straight up towards the sky with your palms touching. As you inhale lift your hips and curl your tailbone upwards. As you exhale and lift your head and chest and press your belly button towards your spine. Reach through your arms and hands. Hold for 3–5 seconds and release. Repeat 3–5 times.

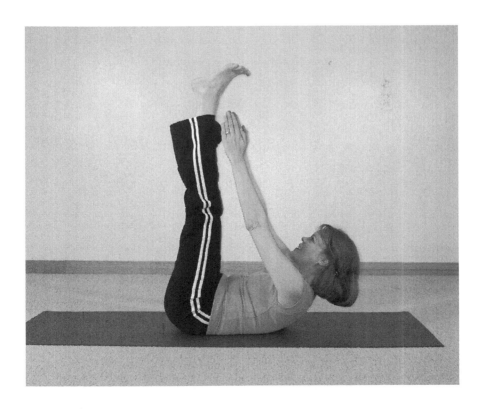

Reverse crunch - legs spread
Level: challenging

Begin by lying on your back. Bring your knees into your chest and extend your legs up towards the ceiling and spread them wide. Extend your arms straight up towards the sky with your palms touching. As you inhale curl your tailbone upwards. As you exhale and lift your head and chest and press your belly button towards your spine. Reach through your arms and hands. Hold for 3–5 seconds and release. Repeat 3–5 times.

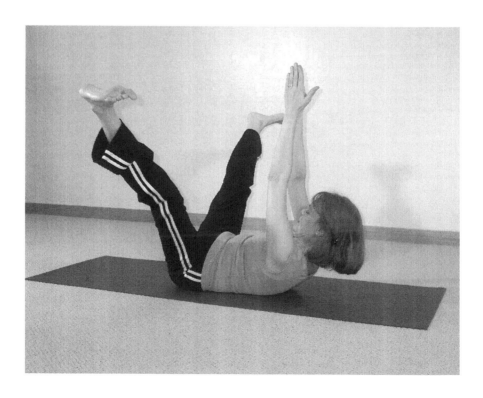

Cross leg crunch
Level: challenging

Begin by lying on your back. As you bring your knees into your chest, cross your right leg over your left. Interlace your fingers behind your head with elbows out at the side. As you exhale lift your torso and head towards your knees. Repeat 3–5 times and then switch the position of your legs. Repeat the exercise on this side. For a variation change leg positions after each time you come up.

Note: The further you move your legs away from your torso the more challenging this exercise becomes.

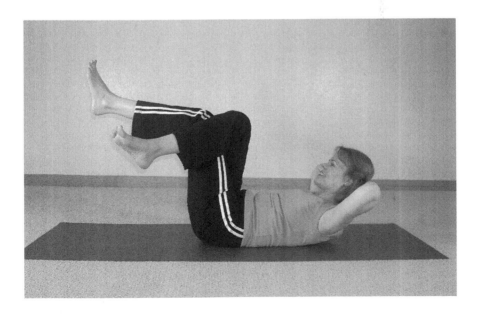

Yoga sit-ups
Level: easy

Begin by lying on your back with knees bent and feet
on floor. Place your hands at the top of your thighs just
under your knees. As you exhale press your belly button
towards the floor and reach your hands towards your
knees, bring your head towards your chest and lift your
torso. Hold for a couple of seconds, then release all the
way to the floor. Repeat 3–5 times.

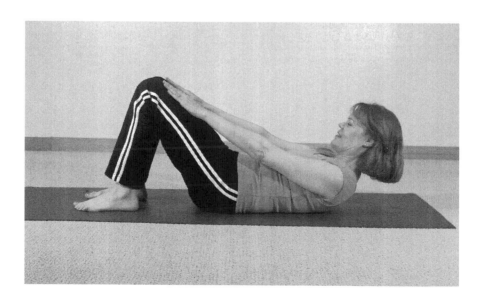

Yoga sit-ups to the side
Level: easy

Begin by lying on your back with knees bent and feet on floor. Place your left hand along side of your left hip and brig your right hand to the top of your left thigh. As you exhale reach your right hand towards your left knee, bringing your head towards your chest and lift your torso. Hold for a couple of seconds, release back to the floor. Repeat 3–5 times and do the other side.

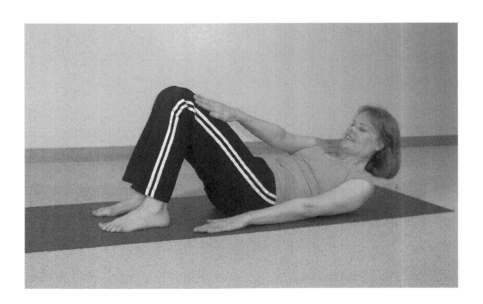

Yoga sit-up with one knee bent
Level: moderate

Begin by lying on your back with your left leg extended
and your right knee bent. Extend your arms straight so
that your hands are along side of your hips. As you
exhale press your belly button towards the floor and lift
your torso reaching your hands towards your left foot.
Hold for a second or two and release to the floor. Repeat
3–5 times and then do the other side.

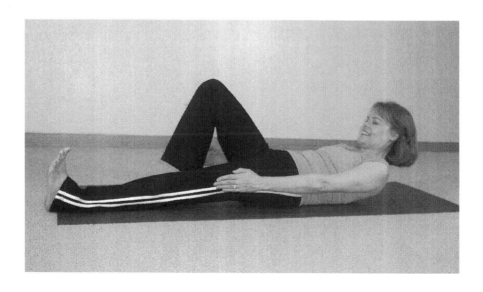

Yoga sit-up with both legs extended
Level: moderate

Begin by lying on your back with both legs extended.
Lift your right leg three inches off ground and extend
arms and hands to towards your feet. As you exhale
press your belly button towards the floor and lift your
torso, reaching your hands towards your feet. Hold for a
second or two and release to the floor. Repeat 3–5 times
and then do the other side.

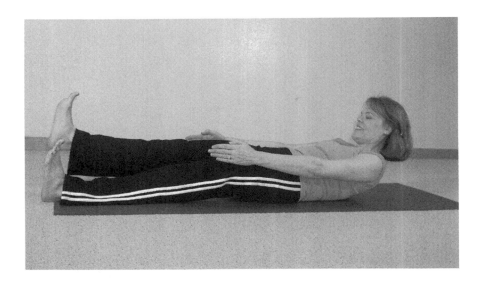

Bicycle
Level: moderate to challenging

Lying on your back bring your knees into your chest
and place your hands behind your head with fingers
touching. Press your bellybutton towards the floor and
bring your right elbow and left knee together. Extend the
right leg straight (about 8–12 inches above the floor.)
Now bring the left elbow and right knee together and
extend the left leg. Repeat the entire sequence 5–10
times.

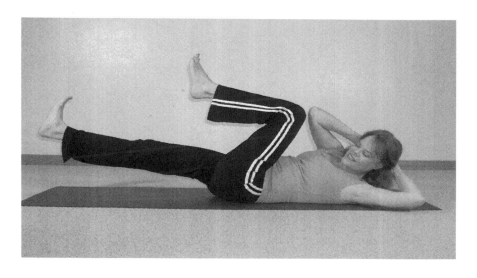

Doggy wag
Level: easy

Starting in table position, you will be on all fours—
knees under hips and hands directly under shoulders.
As you exhale bring your right hip and the right side of
your head towards each other—creating the shape of
the letter C with your torso. Release, and inhale towards
center. Exhale, and bring your left hip and left side of
your head towards each other. Inhale and come back to
center. Repeat the whole sequence 5–7 times. Be sure
to move your hips towards the side of your head that is
turning—not away from your head. This exercise is
particularly good at working the muscles on the sides
of your torso which are called the obliques.

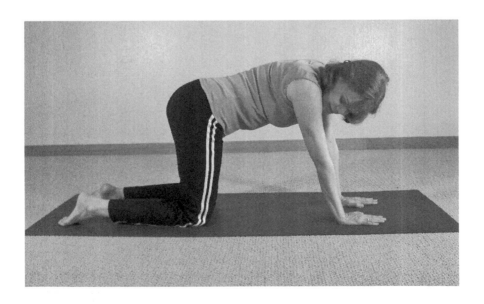

Cat tuck and dog tilt
Level: easy

To prepare for this posture come into table position on all fours—knees under hips and hands directly under shoulders. As you exhale bring you head and hips towards each other and your belly button towards your spine—your back should be arched. Pause there for a second or two. Then inhale, turn your hips forward, and lift your tailbone and your head. Be sure not to overextend you neck. Repeat the whole sequence slowly, 5–7 times.

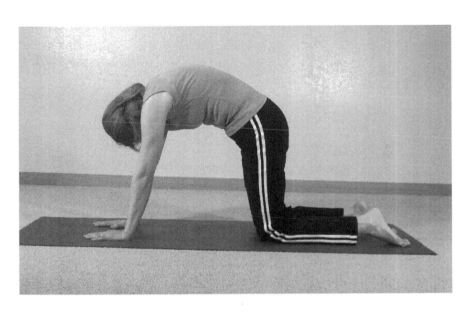

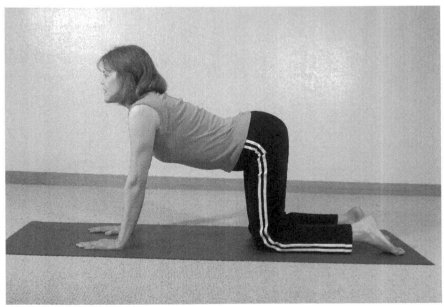

Cat extension
Level: easy

First come into table position on all fours—knees
under hips and hands directly under shoulders. As you
exhale bring your right knee and head towards each
other. Inhale and extend your right leg straight back
behind you as you lift your torso at the same time.
Repeat 5 times and the do the other side.

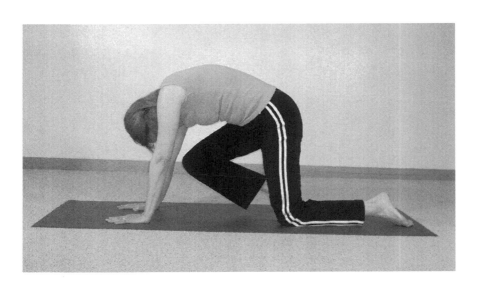

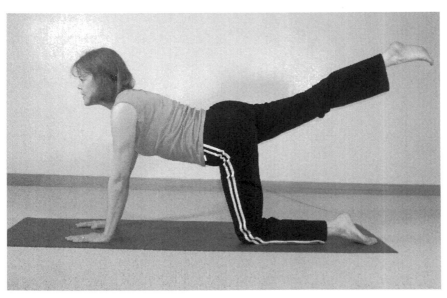

Cat balance
Level: easy

Come into table position on all fours—knees under hips and hands directly under shoulders. Extend your right leg back and then your left arm out in front of you. Hold for 5 long breaths and then do the other side. As a variation switch from side to side holding each side for one breath.

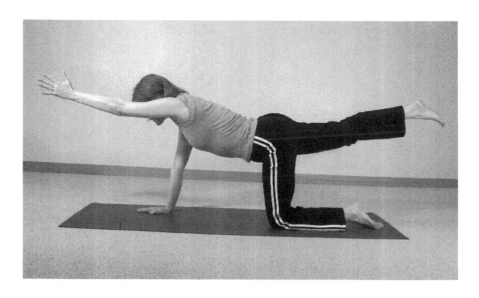

Extended Table
Level: moderate

Come into table position with arms under your
shoulders and knees under your hips. Walk your hands
forward about six inches so that your arms are in front
of your shoulders. Extend your right arm forward
and take 5 breaths. Release and do the other side. For
more intensity let your torso and hips come forward
a little more.

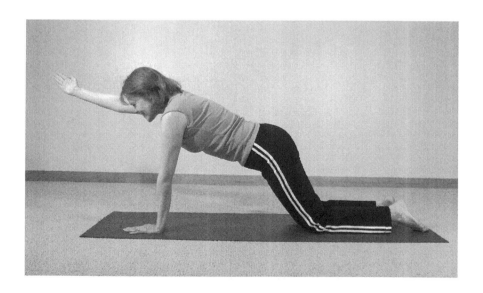

Plank
Level: moderate

Start by coming onto your hands and knees in table position. Make sure your arms are right under your shoulders and your fingers are pointing straight ahead. Now walk your feet backwards into plank (high push up position). You want your torso, hips and legs all in one line—don't let your hips drop or lift too high. Press your hands into the floor and lift up into your shoulders. Take your bellybutton towards your spine and stretch through your heels. Work up to holding for a slow count of 10. This exercise is good for your arms and upper body as well as your abs!

Note: If your upper body is challenged in this exercise you can make it easier by coming onto your knees until you build the strength to perform it with your legs extended off the ground.

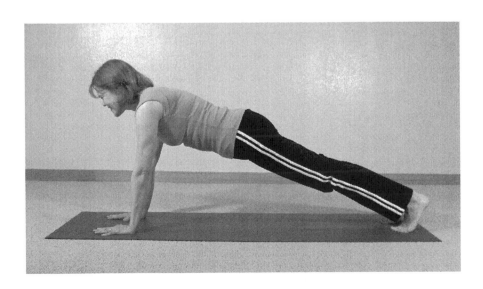

Plank with one leg off the ground
Level: moderate

Start by coming onto your hands and knees in table position. Make sure your arms are right under your shoulders and your fingers are pointing straight ahead. Now walk your feet backwards into plank (high push up position). You want your torso, hips and legs all in one line—don't let your hips drop or lift too high. Press your hands into the floor and lift up into your shoulders. Take your bellybutton towards your spine and stretch through your heels. Now lift your right leg off the ground so it is parallel to the floor. Hold for a slow count of 5 and then release your right foot to the floor. Repeat the exercise on your left side.

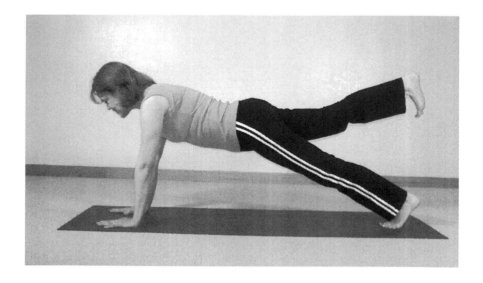

Plank with one arm
Level: challenging

Start by coming onto your hands and knees in table position. Make sure your arms are right under your shoulders and your fingers are pointing straight ahead. Now walk your feet backwards into plank (high push up position). You want your torso, hips and legs all in one line—don't let your hips drop or lift too high. Press hands into the floor and lift up into your shoulders. Take your bellybutton towards your spine and stretch through your heels. Now extend your right arm directly out in front of you. Keep your hips level. Hold for a slow count of 5 and then release your right foot to the floor. Repeat the exercise on your left side.

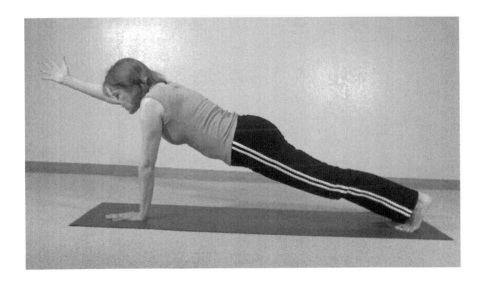

Flying Plank
Level: challenging (very!)

Start by coming onto your hands and knees in table position. Make sure your arms are right under your shoulders and your fingers are pointing straight ahead. Now walk your feet backwards into plank (high push up position). You want your torso, hips and legs all in one line—don't let your hips drop or lift too high. Press your hands into the floor and lift up into your shoulders. Take your bellybutton towards your spine and stretch through your heels. Now lift your right leg off the ground so it is parallel to the floor and at the same time extend your left arm directly out in front of you. Keep your hips level. Hold for a slow count of 5 and then release your right foot to the floor and left hand to the floor. Repeat the exercise on you're the other side with your left leg and right arm.

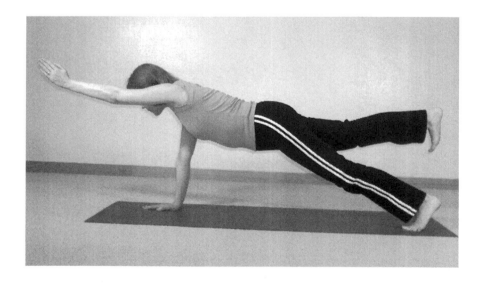

Side crunch with leg lift

Level: easy

Begin by lying on your right side, bend your right elbow so that your right hand supports your head. Make sure that your legs, hips, torso, shoulder and extended elbow are all in one line. Press through both heels and lift your left leg as high as possible. Hold for 5–8 breaths and release. Do the other side.

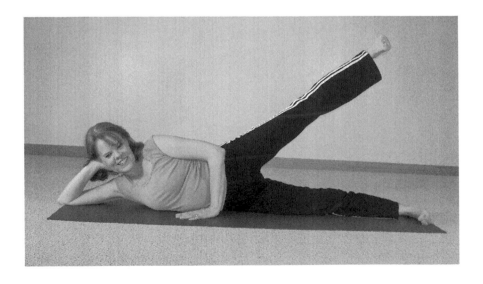

Side crunch with two legs
Level: moderate

Begin by lying on your right side, bend your right elbow so that your right hand supports your head. Make sure that your legs, hips, torso, shoulder and extended elbow are all in one line. Press through both heels and lift both legs off the ground. Hold for 5–8 breaths and release. Do the other side.

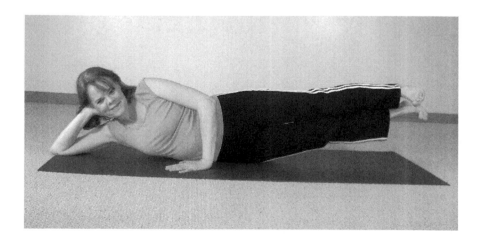

Side crunch—leg to leg
Level: moderate

Begin by lying on your right side, bend your right elbow so that your right hand supports your head. Make sure that your legs, hips, torso, shoulder and extended elbow are all in one line. Press through both heels and lift your left leg as high as possible. Now take your right leg up to meet you left. You may need to lower the left slightly to accomplish this. Hold for 5–8 breaths and release. Do the other side.

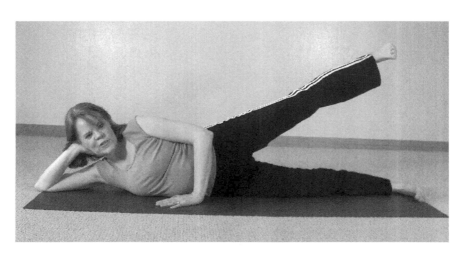

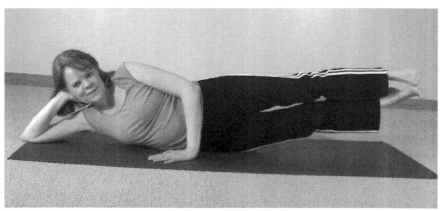

Side crunch with chest lift
Level: challenging

Begin by lying on your right side, make sure that your legs, hips, torso, and shoulder are all in one line. Cross your arms across your chest. Press through both heels. Lift both legs up towards the ceiling as you lift the right side of your torso off the floor. Point your left shoulder towards your left foot, squeezing the left side of your abdomen. Hold for 5–8 breaths and release. Repeat on the other side.

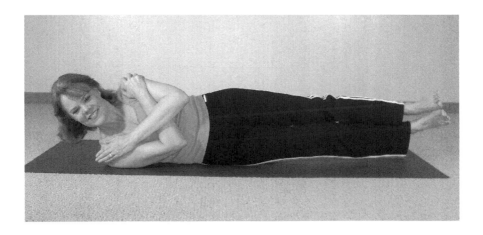

Arm bar with foot over foot
Level: challenging

To begin bring your right hip on the floor and extend your right leg directly from your right hip. Extend your left leg directly over your right with the inner feet touching. Next extend your right arm at a bit of an angle in front of your right shoulder. Now, press through both heels and into the right hand to lift off the floor. Reach strongly through your left arm and squeeze right side oblique muscles (on the side of your torso) as you lift your hips. Work up to a slow count of five and come down. Repeat on other side.

If you need to make this exercise a little easier bring your top foot onto the floor in front of your bottom leg knee.

In addition to working the obliques this exercise is very good for building strength in the arms and upper body.

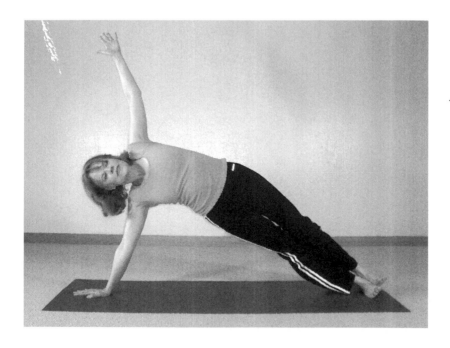

Arm bar
Level: moderate

To begin bring your right hip on the floor and extend your right leg directly from your right hip. Place your left foot on the floor directly in front of your right knee. Next extend your right arm is at a bit of an angle in front of your right shoulder. Press into your right hand and both feet and lift your hips up towards the sky. Reach strongly through your left arm and squeeze right side oblique muscles (on the side of your torso) as you lift your hips. Work up to a slow count of five and come down. Repeat on other side.

In addition to working the obliques this exercise is very good for building strength in the arms and upper body.

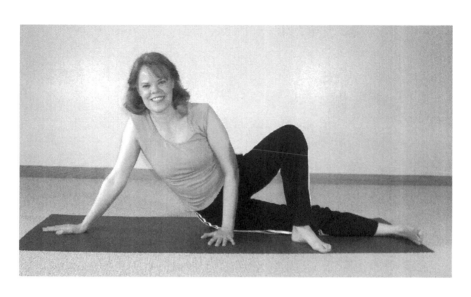

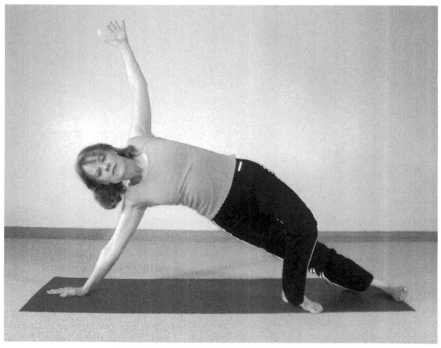

Toe touch
Level: moderate

Begin by lying on your back, bring your knees into towards your chest. Slowly release your feet towards the floor so that only your toes touch. Once your toes touch bring your knees back towards your chest—go slowly. Repeat 5–8 times.

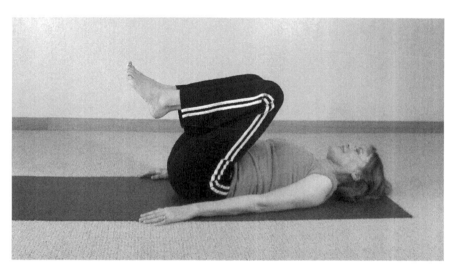

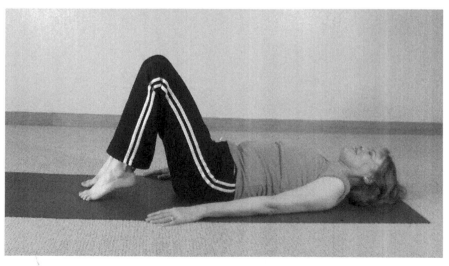

Alternating toe touch
Level: moderate

Begin by lying on your back, bring your knees into towards your chest. Slowly release your left foot towards the floor so that only your toes touch. Bring your left knee into your chest and let the toes of the right foot touch the floor. Go back and forth from side to side. Repeat the cycle several times.

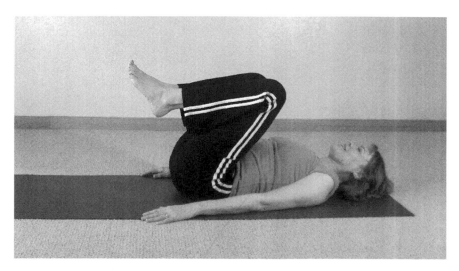

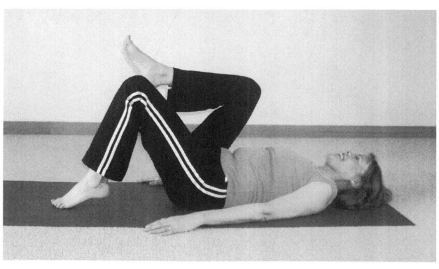

Leg release with bent knee
Level: easy

Begin by lying on your back with knees bent and feet on the floor. Bring your arms overhead, behind you. Reach through your fingertips. Extend your right leg up towards the sky. Reaching through your right foot, slowly release your right leg 2–3 inches from the floor. Slowly take you leg back up. Repeat 2–3 times on the right side and then do the left side.

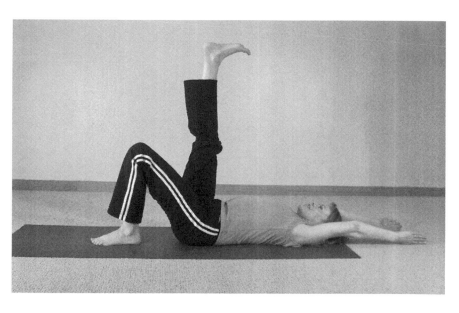

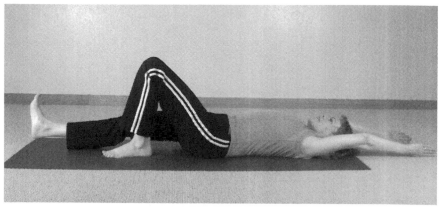

Leg release with straight legs
Level: moderate

Begin by lying on your back, bring your arms overhead
behind you, and reach through your fingertips. Bring
your knees into your chest and then extend both legs to
towards the ceiling. Continue to reach through both feet
as you slowly lower your right leg 2–3 inches from the
floor and then slowly bring it back up. Repeat 2–3 times
and then do the left side.

Note: If at any time you feel pain in your back bend
your knee and come out of the exercise. Try doing the
exercise with releasing your leg only half way to the
floor. If you are still feeling discomfort in your back
don't do the exercise.

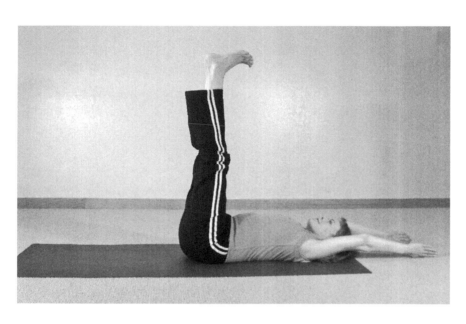

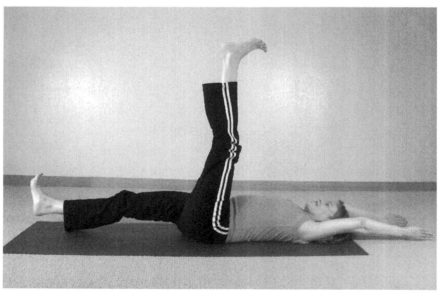

Leg release with two legs
Level: challenging

Begin by lying on your back, bring your arms overhead,
behind you, and reach through your fingertips. Bring
your knees into your chest and then extend both legs to
towards the ceiling. Continue to reach through both feet
as you slowly lower both legs 2–3 inches from the floor.
Repeat as many times as you can. For more challenge in
this exercise release your legs towards the floor in steps,
release about 12 inches at a time and waiting a few
seconds before dropping your legs to the next level.

Note: If at any time you feel pain in your back bend
your knees and come out of the exercise. Try doing the
exercise with releasing your legs only half way to the
floor. If you are still feeling discomfort in your back
don't do the exercise.

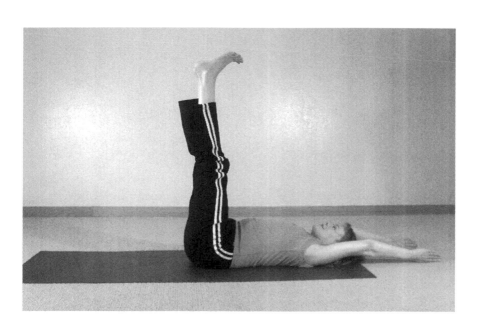

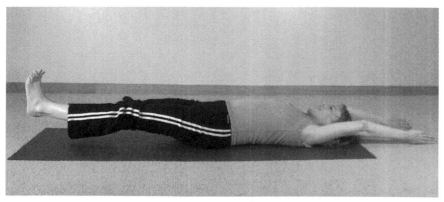

Tracing the floor
Level: challenging

Begin by lying on your back, bring your arms overhead behind you, and reach through your fingertips. Bring your knees into your chest and then extend both legs to towards the ceiling. Continue to reach through both feet as you slowly lower both legs 2–3 inches from the floor. Keeping your feet 2–3 inches off the ground, slowly bend your knees as you trace your heels above the floor. When your heels are close to your hips, bring your knees into your chest and extend your legs. Repeat 3–5 times. Now reverse the direction. Start with your legs extended 2–3 inches off the ground and lift them up towards the ceiling so they are at a right angle to your torso. Bend your knees and trace your heels just above the floor until your legs are straight. Repeat 3–5 times.

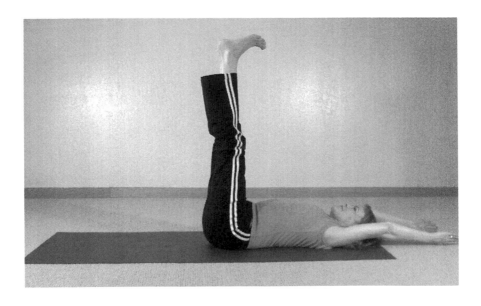

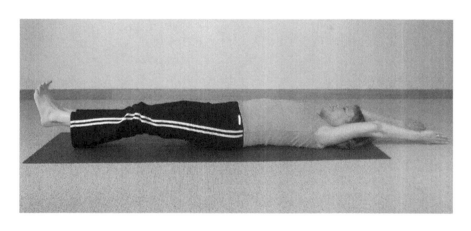

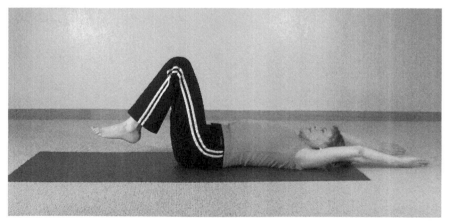

Knee down twist
Level: easy

Begin by lying on your back and extend your arms from your shoulders making a T position with your torso. Move your hips a couple inches to the right. Bring your knees into your chest and then take them up and over to the left—to the floor. Look back to your right hand. Take 5 to 10 breaths and then repeat on the other side. For more challenge, extend your legs straight towards your hand once you are in the twist.

Note: Don't force your knees to the floor if they don't touch. Instead put something under your knees—such as a folded blanket, a pillow or some books.

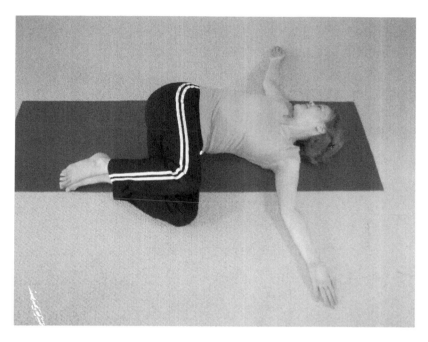

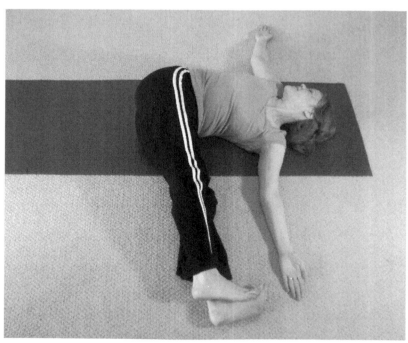

Knee down twist—side to side
Level: moderate

Begin by lying on your back, extend your arms from your shoulders making a T position with your torso. Bring your knees into your chest and drop them to your right as you exhale. Inhale and bring your knees to center, exhale and release them to the left. Inhale them up to center and exhale them to the right. Continue going back and forth for several rounds.

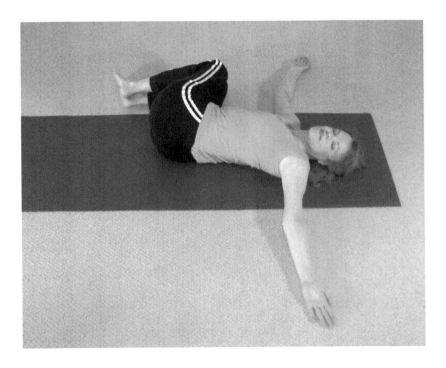

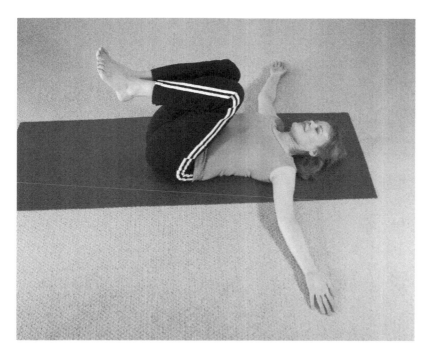

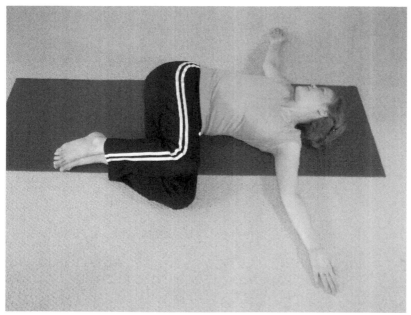

Belly Turner
Level: challenging

Begin by lying on your back, move your hips a couple inches to the right. Extend your arms to the sides and bring your knees into your chest. Extend your legs toward the ceiling and then take both feet towards your left hand. Once your feet touch the floor bring them closer to your left hand - continue to press through both heels. Take 5 to 10 breaths. Take your legs up and do the other side.

If it is hard to control your legs or you feel pain in your back, then bend your knees to lower or raise your legs. Be sure to straighten your legs when they are on the floor facing your hand.

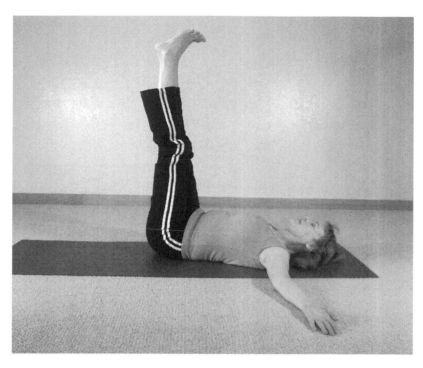

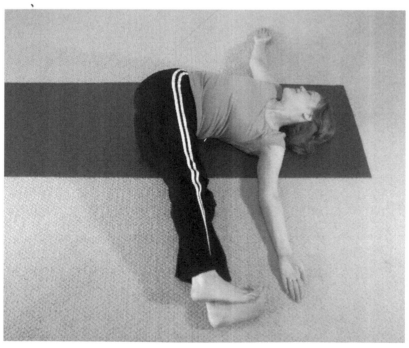

Bridge
Level: easy

Begin by lying on the floor, bend your knees and place your feet on the floor. Have you legs in line with your hips and your feet under your knees. Bring your arms along side of your hips, reaching towards your feet with the palms facing down. As you inhale press into your arms and feet as you lift your hips towards the ceiling. Exhale as your release your hips to the floor. Repeat 5–8 times.

Note: If you suffer from lower back issues, be careful in this posture as well as other variations of Bridge. If you feel pain in your lower back, avoid the Bridge posture.

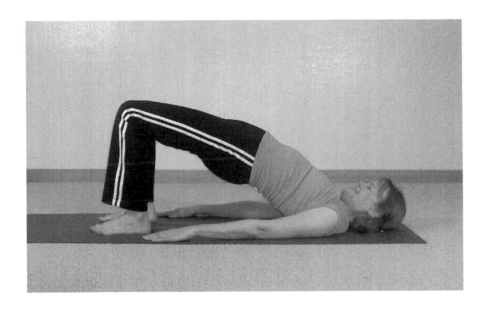

Single leg bridge
Level: moderate

Begin by lying on the floor, bend your knees and place
your feet on the floor. Have you legs in line with your
hips and your feet under your knees. Bring your arms
along side of your hips, reaching towards your feet with
the palms facing down. Cross your right ankle onto your
left thigh. As you inhale press into your arms and left
foot as you lift your hips off the floor. Exhale to come
down. Repeat 5–8 times and then do the other side. As a
variation change the leg crossing after each complete up
and down cycle.

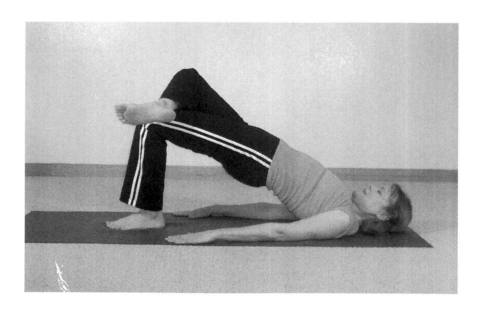

Bridge with knee into chest
Level: moderate

Begin by lying on the floor, bend your knees and place your feet on the floor. Have your legs in line with your hips and your feet under your knees. Bring your arms along side of your hips, reaching towards your feet with the palms facing down. Bring your right knee into towards your chest and interlace your fingers behind your right thigh. As you inhale press your left foot into the floor and lift your hips. Exhale and come down. Repeat 5–8 times and then do the other side. As a variation have your arms on the floor. Press into your arms and left foot as you lift your hips off the floor. Exhale to come down.

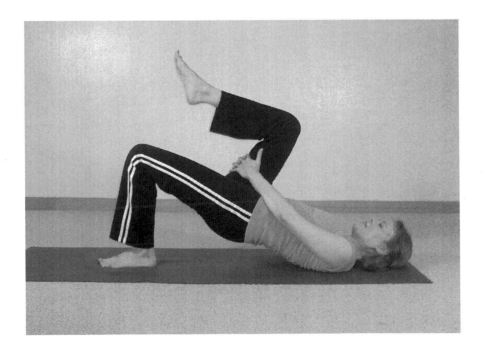

Cooling down

Now that your abdominal muscles have been worked, you have most likely spent a lot of time contracting them. To help them and you relax it is a good idea to stretch them out.

Lie on your back with legs extended. Take your arms overhead behind you. As you inhale reach through your fingertips and your heels. As you exhale release the stretch. Repeat several times. Focus on your breath—making you belly big on the inhale and releasing on the exhale. Once you are through with this cool down exercise, rest for a couple minutes on the floor before getting up.

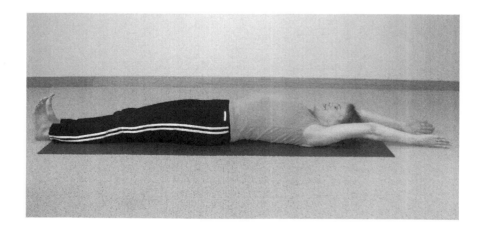

List of exercises by challenge level

Easy

Moderate

Challenging

Has this book been helpful to you?

If so, please consider leaving a positive review on Amazon so others may be helped as well. If on the other hand, you feel this book needs to be changed or added to in some way please let us know so that we can make those changes. Email: info@letsdoyoga.com

Ageless Beauty & Timeless Strength.
A woman's guide to building upper body strength without any special equipment.

Learn how to dramatically reduce the risk of modern diseases and improve longevity without pills diets or creams.

Discover the life affirming benefits of fun body-weight only exercises to: Lose weight while becoming stronger & more toned! Sleep better & become healthier overall! Experience more self - confidence and look & feel your best! Have more energy & enhanced sense of well-being!

Discover one of the most important keys for longevity & why health experts are extremely excited about resistance training. Reverse osteoporosis: Strength training can stop the loss of bone AND increase bone bass by up to 9% within a year. Lose and maintain weight - stop yo-yo dieting. Reduce the risk of type 2 diabetes. Slow and prevent arthritis. Significantly reduce your risk of heart disease & high blood pressure. Could this be the fountain of youth? You decide!

Learn cutting edge nutrition secrets for maximizing strength & energy. Maximize your workouts to get the most benefits in the least amount of time. Fun, interesting, & challenging exercises for all levels.

Also included are inspiring biographies of women who use strength training to improve and positively impact their lives.

Visit www.amazon.com to order

Beginning Yoga: A Practice Manual

An essential resource for beginning through intermediate yoga students! *Beginning Yoga: A Practice Manual* has been carefully designed to help students develop a solid foundation in yoga through their home practice.

This is a clearly written, easy to use book with just the right amount of information to support your practice. And it's large 8 1/2 X 11 format makes it easy to use. A thoughtful balance of theory and practice are presented to provide you with a context as well as instruction for your practice.

Features:

- Fifty postures detailed with full page photos and clear step-by-step instructions
- Intro to meditation
- Intro to pranayama (yogic breathing)
- Over 20 follow along practice sessions with words and pictures.
- Specific practices for energy, relaxation, and preventative back care.
- Lay flat book binding stays open for easy reference.

Visit www.amazon.com to order

Release Your Shoulders, Relax Your Neck
The best exercises for releasing shoulder tension and neck pain.

Do you suffer from tight shoulders, upper back, or neck area? *Tight Shoulder Relief* is a must! Learn why your shoulders get tight, shows you how to effectively relieve them, improve flexibility, and prevent future problems.

Get ready to feel good in your body again! Ideal for computer users, dental hygienists, hair stylists, athletes, massage therapists and anyone who carries a lot of stress in their shoulders. This is the only book solely dedicated to helping your relieve tight shoulder problems!

Features: Over 50 exercises to relieve tight shoulders. Photos of exercises with easy to follow directions. Shoulder anatomy 101. How your shoulders move and why they get so tight. Additional tips for relieving tight shoulders.

Visit www.amazon.com to order.

GERD & Acid Reflux Solutions
Your guide to prevention, treatment, cures, & relief!

Do you suffer from heartburn or perhaps one of the other uncomfortable symptoms of GERD, also known as "acid reflux" including:

Unexplained chest pain	Abdominal pain
Difficulty swallowing	Unexplained weight loss
Excessive burping & belching	Dental decay
Frequent nausea & vomiting	Passing of black stool
Persistent coughing or hoarseness	Wheezing or asthma-type symptoms

Laryngitis, sinusitis or ear infections

And if the physical symptoms of GERD weren't bad enough, you may also lack the joy of eating and socializing, have trouble sleeping, face economic hardship, suffer anxiety associated with medical procedures, and have a reduction in the quality of life.

Linked to advanced stages of GERD is esophageal cancer - the fasting growing cancer diagnosis in the U.S., with prevalence doubling in the last 10 years. *Just as alarming is that GERD has reached epidemic proportions with 1 of every 4 people afflicted by it.*

This book explains why GERD has become so prevalent, provides clear understanding of what is happening inside your body when GERD is

present, and gives you with the insight and tools to prevent, reverse and manage this illness so you can feel good again.

In "GERD & Acid Reflux Solutions" you will discover:

- How to identify risk factors & warning signs so you can take charge of your health before complications arise.

- Effective prevention strategies.

- How to significantly reduce or eliminate symptoms of GERD with natural alternative treatments such as herbs & supplements as well as easy to make lifestyle adjustments.

- Medical interventions: Prescription and non-prescription medications - how they work and their side effects. And if needed, surgical options are also discussed.

- Which foods aggravate GERD, and which foods are soothing and improve digestion, along with sample recipes that are healthy, delicious and soothing.

Regardless of the severity of your GERD, this book will guide you to end the suffering of GERD and improve your overall health and well-being.

How can I get to sleep?
Your guide to overcoming insomnia, sleeplessness, and getting a good night sleep.

Not sleeping can be a nightmare! Lying awake, tossing and turning, mental agitations and the exhaustion that follows are definitely not a party! The side effects of insomnia and not be able to sleep can reduce your productivity, make you moody and irritable, and lead to numerous physical ailments including obesity, hypertension, lack of coordination, weight gain, etc.

In *Insomnia Cures* you'll discover the **secrets of sleeping like a baby:**

- Uncover what is really keeping you up at night; the answer might surprise you!
- Get the best **non-drug methods for getting to sleep naturally** with our "Insomnia Tool Box."
- Create healthy sleeping habits so you **sleep well night after night**.
- How to **get back to sleep** when you wake up in the middle of the night.
- **Reduce and eliminate tension and anxiety** with powerful stress management techniques that help quiet your mind, remove stress from your body, and slip easily into a good night's sleep.
- How to **eat your way to a good night sleep**: which foods actually help you fall asleep and which will keep you from falling asleep.
- *Special section:* gentle yoga postures and breathing practices that are deeply relaxing, helping you **get to sleep sooner and sleep longer**. Instructions and photos included.

Bonus audios worth $9.95: (link to audio download provided in book) 1. *Progressive Relaxation*: a proven method for reducing anxiety, eliminating stress and helping you get to sleep - particularly helpful if you wake in the middle of the night. Having this audio makes it easier to just listen instead having to talk yourself back to sleep

Don't spend another sleepless night tossing and turning when you can sleep well tonight. In this book you'll find everything you need to **say good night to insomnia forever!**

Visit www.amazon.com to order

Meditation: The Gift Inside.
How to meditate to quiet your mind, find inner peace and lasting happiness

For thousands of years people of faith, ascetics as well as everyday people have practiced meditation to quiet their minds, find inner peace and connect with their spirit.

Whether you are looking for a book on meditation for beginners or you are an experienced meditator wanting to renew your practice you'll find "Meditation: The Gift Inside" connects you to the heart of the practice. This meditation book covers:

- How to meditate like a yogi: experience the same meditation techniques that the deepest meditators use.

- Uncover the secrets to quiet your mind; have inner peace even when your outer world may be chaotic.

- Powerful methods to dramatically deepen your meditation.

- How to easily make meditation a part of your daily life and eliminate challenges that may prevent you from practicing regularly.

- Discover how modern scientific research is confirming what the ancient yogis knew about the extraordinary benefits of meditation including: sleeping better, reducing pain, improving mood, extending life, etc.

- Explore the connection between yoga and meditation.

Visit www.amazon.com to order

Office Ergonomics: Preventing Repetitive
Motion Injuries & Carpal Tunnel Syndrome

If your profession involves working at a computer or a requires repetitive motion then the probability that you will experience an injury is very high. Perhaps you are already experiencing symptoms such as tingling, pain, tightness or numbness in your wrist, elbow, shoulder, neck, or back.

The good news is that there is a lot you can to do to prevent, eliminate and reduce the possibility of injury. Office Ergonomics is the only book available to offer comprehensive solutions for avoiding and reducing costly, painful, and debilitating injuries. If you spend more than 1 hour per day on a computer you need this book - there is no need to risk injury or be in pain any longer!

Features:

- 100's of tips for making your workstation comfortable, efficient and for reducing the risk of injury.

- Causes and treatment of repetitive motion injuries.

- Positions and setups you must avoid.

- Fixes that don t work.

- Behavioral prevention tips.

- How ergonomics helps.

- Bonus: Exercises to relieve stress at computer & workstations.

Visit www.amazon.com to order

Notes

Notes

Notes

Notes